Augmentin

Discover the Healing Power of an Antibiotic for Infections such as Urinary Tract, Respiratory Tract, Ear, Sinuses, and Skin Infections

Andy Stewart

Table of Contents

CHAPTER ONE

Understanding the Benefits of Augmentin for Treating Bacterial Infections

Augmentin is an antibiotic medication used to treat a variety of bacterial infections. It is a combination of two drugs, amoxicillin and clavulanate potassium, which work together to inhibit the activity of certain bacteria. The combination of these two medications is effective in treating a wide range of bacterial infections, including those of the skin, sinuses, ears, and lungs.

The first medication, amoxicillin, is a penicillin-type antibiotic that works by inhibiting the production of bacterial cell walls. By preventing the formation of the cell walls, amoxicillin makes it difficult for the bacteria to survive and reproduce. Clavulanate potassium is an inhibitor of beta-lactamase enzymes, which are produced naturally by some bacteria. Beta-lactamase enzymes can break down the amoxicillin, rendering it ineffective. By inhibiting these enzymes, clavulanate potassium prevents this breakdown, allowing the amoxicillin to remain effective against the bacteria.

The combination of amoxicillin and clavulanate potassium is used to treat a wide variety of bacterial infections, including skin infections, such as impetigo, abscesses, and cellulitis; sinus infections; ear infections; and lung infections.

Augmentin is also effective in treating certain urinary tract infections, such as cystitis, and can be used to prevent certain infections, such as endocarditis. In addition, Augmentin may be used to treat certain sexually transmitted infections, such as gonorrhea and chlamydia.

There are several benefits to using Augmentin to treat bacterial infections. First, it is effective against a wide range of bacteria, making it an appropriate choice for treating many types of infections. Second, it is easy to administer, as it is available in several forms, including tablets, oral suspension, and chewable tablets. Third, the combination of amoxicillin and clavulanate potassium provides excellent coverage against beta-lactamase-producing bacteria, making it effective against certain bacteria that are resistant to other types of antibiotics.

In addition, Augmentin has a low risk of side effects. The most common side effect is diarrhea, which is usually mild and can be managed with appropriate diet and hydration. Other side effects are rare, but may include headaches, rash, nausea, vomiting, and abdominal pain. However, Augmentin is generally well tolerated and can be used safely by most people.

Overall, Augmentin is an effective antibiotic for treating a wide range of bacterial infections. It is easy to administer, has a low risk of side effects, and provides excellent coverage against beta-lactamase-producing bacteria. For these reasons, it is an appropriate choice for treating many types of bacterial infections.

What is Augmentin and How Does It Work?

Augmentin is an antibiotic that is commonly used to treat bacterial infections. It is a combination of two different antibiotics, amoxicillin and clavulanic acid, that work together to kill bacteria and stop their growth. The amoxicillin works by inhibiting the growth of bacteria, while the clavulanic acid works by preventing the bacteria from breaking down the amoxicillin, allowing it to be effective against a wider range of bacteria.

Augmentin is used to treat a wide range of bacterial infections, including bronchitis, sinusitis, tonsillitis, skin infections, urinary tract infections, and ear infections. It can also be used to prevent infection after a surgery. Augmentin is usually taken orally, but can also be given in liquid form or injection.

When taken properly, Augmentin can be effective in treating bacterial infections. It is important to note that it does not work against viral infections, such as the common cold or flu. It is also important to finish the entire course of treatment, even if the symptoms of the infection have gone away. This helps to ensure that all of the bacteria are killed and the infection does not come back.

The most common side effects of Augmentin include nausea, vomiting, diarrhea, and headache. If these side effects occur, it is important to contact a doctor right away. In some cases, Augmentin can cause an allergic reaction, which may include rash, hives, itching, or difficulty breathing. If you experience any of these symptoms, it is important to stop taking Augmentin and seek medical help right away.

It is important to take Augmentin exactly as prescribed by your doctor. This will help to ensure that the medication is effective in treating the infection. If you miss a dose, it is important to take it as soon as you remember, but if it is almost time for your next dose, skip the missed dose and continue on your regular dosing schedule. Taking too much of the medication can increase your risk of side effects.

Augmentin is a powerful antibiotic and it is important to take it exactly as prescribed. If you experience any side effects or if you think that the medication is not working, it is important to contact your doctor right away. They will be able to adjust your dose or prescribe a different antibiotic if needed. Augmentin can be a very effective treatment for bacterial infections, when taken as directed.

CHAPTER TWO

Augmentin: An Overview of Side Effects and Interactions

Augmentin is an antibiotic that is commonly prescribed to treat a wide range of bacterial infections, including bronchitis, sinusitis, and pneumonia. It is a combination of amoxicillin and clavulanate potassium, and is effective against some bacteria that are resistant to other antibiotics. While it is generally considered safe and effective, there are some side effects and interactions associated with Augmentin that patients should be aware of.

One of the most common side effects of Augmentin is an upset stomach. This may manifest as nausea, vomiting, diarrhea, or abdominal cramping. Additionally, patients may experience a mild rash or hives. These side effects usually resolve on their own and do not require medical attention. More severe reactions, such as difficulty breathing, swelling of the face and throat, or anaphylaxis, are rare but require immediate medical attention.

Augmentin can also interact with other medications, including anticoagulants, nonsteroidal anti-inflammatory drugs, and certain antidepressants. It is important for patients to tell their healthcare provider about all medications they are taking, as well as any supplements, to ensure that there are no interactions. Additionally, Augmentin can cause altered results on certain laboratory tests, such as those that measure liver or kidney function.

Due to its potential to interact with other medications, Augmentin should not be taken with antacids or iron supplements. It also should not be taken with alcohol, as it can increase the risk of side effects. Additionally, patients should avoid using Augmentin if they have a history of liver disease, kidney disease, mononucleosis, or a history of allergic reactions to penicillin or other antibiotics.

Finally, pregnant women should not take Augmentin without consulting their healthcare provider, as it may cause harm to the unborn baby. This is especially true in the first trimester, as Augmentin has been linked to birth defects. Women who are breastfeeding should also discuss the risks and benefits of taking Augmentin with their healthcare provider.

In summary, Augmentin is an effective antibiotic for treating many bacterial infections. However, it is important for patients to be aware of the potential side effects and interactions associated with this medication. Patients should always consult their healthcare provider before taking Augmentin, and should not take it with antacids, iron supplements, alcohol, or other medications without first consulting their healthcare provider. Additionally, pregnant women and those who are breastfeeding should discuss the risks and benefits of taking Augmentin with their healthcare provider before starting the medication. By being aware of the potential side effects and interactions associated with Augmentin, patients can make an informed decision about whether this medication is right for them.

How to Take Augmentin and Ensure Maximum Effectiveness

Taking Augmentin (amoxicillin/clavulanate) is an important step in the treatment of a variety of bacterial infections. While it can be effective at treating the condition, it is important to take this medication properly in order to ensure maximum effectiveness. Here are some tips on how to take Augmentin and ensure maximum effectiveness:

1. Follow your doctor's instructions. Your doctor will provide you with specific instructions on how to take Augmentin. This may include the dosage, as well as the frequency and duration of use. Be sure to follow your doctor's instructions to the letter in order to ensure maximum effectiveness.

2. Take the medication with a full glass of water. Augmentin should always be taken

with a full glass of water, as this helps to ensure that it is absorbed properly into your system.

3. Take the medication at the same time each day. Taking Augmentin at the same time each day helps to ensure that the medication remains in your system at a consistent level. This helps to maximize the effectiveness of the medication.

4. Do not skip doses. Missing doses of Augmentin can reduce its effectiveness, as the medication may not remain in your system at a consistent level. If you forget to take a dose, take it as soon as you remember. However, do not take two

doses at once, as this can increase the risk of side effects.

5. Do not take Augmentin with dairy products. Dairy products can interfere with the absorption of the medication, reducing its effectiveness.

6. Do not take Augmentin with antacids. Antacids can reduce the effectiveness of the medication by preventing it from being absorbed properly.

7. Do not take Augmentin with other medications. Taking Augmentin with other medications can increase the risk of side

effects and reduce its effectiveness. Talk to your doctor before taking any other medications while on Augmentin.

8. Store the medication properly. Augmentin should be stored at room temperature and away from light and moisture.

9. Discard any unused medication. Any unused medication should be discarded properly to avoid any potential misuse.

10. Report any side effects. Augmentin can cause a variety of side effects. If you

experience any of these, be sure to report it to your doctor as soon as possible.

By following these tips, you can help ensure that you take Augmentin properly and maximize its effectiveness. Be sure to follow your doctor's instructions and speak to them if you have any questions or concerns. If you experience any side effects, be sure to report them to your doctor right away.

CHAPTER THREE

Augmentin: Dosage Guidelines for Children and Adults

Augmentin is a combination antibiotic that is used to treat a variety of bacterial infections. It contains amoxicillin, a type of penicillin, and clavulanate potassium, which helps prevent certain bacteria from becoming resistant to amoxicillin. It is available in both oral and intravenous forms and is prescribed to treat various infections such as sinusitis, pneumonia, bronchitis, and ear infections. Augmentin is generally safe for use in both children and adults and is often the first-line treatment for bacterial infections.

When considering the use of Augmentin, the dosage and frequency of administration are important factors to consider. The dosage of Augmentin for adults is typically 250 to 500 milligrams (mg) every 8 hours or 500 to 875 mg every 12 hours, depending on the infection being treated. For children, the dose of Augmentin is usually lower. The physician will determine the correct dosage based on the child's weight, age and the type of infection.

Most adults should take Augmentin with or without food every 8 to 12 hours for 7 to 10 days, depending on the type and severity of the infection. The total length of therapy may be extended if the infection is not responding to the treatment. For children, Augmentin is usually given twice daily for 10 days. It is important to finish the full course of the medication, even if the symptoms disappear, in order to completely clear the infection.

It is important to take Augmentin exactly as prescribed by the physician. Taking more than the prescribed dose can lead to serious side effects such as diarrhea, nausea, vomiting and abdominal pain. Taking Augmentin with food can help reduce the risk of stomach upset. It is also important to take Augmentin at the same time each day.

Some people may be allergic to penicillin or have a history of liver or kidney disease. These individuals should not take Augmentin or should be closely monitored while taking the medication. Pregnant and breastfeeding women should consult their doctor before taking Augmentin.

In summary, Augmentin is a combination antibiotic that is used to treat a variety of bacterial infections. It is generally safe for use in both children and adults and is often the first-line treatment for bacterial infections. The dosage of Augmentin for adults is typically 250 to 500 mg every 8 hours or 500 to 875 mg every 12 hours, depending on the infection being treated. For children, the dose of Augmentin is usually lower. Most adults should take

Augmentin with or without food every 8 to 12 hours for 7 to 10 days, depending on the type and severity of the infection. It is important to take Augmentin exactly as prescribed by the physician and to take it at the same time each day. Some people may be allergic to penicillin or have a history of liver or kidney disease, and these individuals should not take Augmentin or should be closely monitored while taking the medication. Pregnant and breastfeeding women should consult their doctor before taking Augmentin.

Pros and Cons of Augmentin Treatment for Bacterial Infections

Augmentin is an antibiotic that contains

two active ingredients, amoxicillin and clavulanic acid, which are used to treat a variety of bacterial infections. Augmentin is a broad-spectrum antibiotic, meaning it is effective against a wide range of bacteria. It is commonly prescribed for respiratory tract infections, urinary tract infections, sinus infections, and other bacterial infections.

The pros of using Augmentin to treat bacterial infections are numerous. It is a safe and effective treatment for many types of bacterial infections. It is also generally well-tolerated and has few side effects. Furthermore, it is a broad-spectrum antibiotic, meaning it is effective against a wide range of bacteria. This makes it a good choice for treating infections caused by multiple bacteria. Additionally, Augmentin can be used to treat infections caused by antibiotic-resistant bacteria, making it a valuable tool in treating serious infections.

However, there are also some potential cons of using Augmentin to treat bacterial infections. The most significant of these is that it is not effective against all types of bacteria. Some bacteria, such as mycoplasma, are not susceptible to the drug. Additionally, Augmentin may be less effective against some types of bacteria, such as Pseudomonas, Enterobacter, and Klebsiella. Additionally, Augmentin can cause side effects, such as nausea, vomiting, and diarrhea. It may also interact with other medications, and it can cause allergic reactions in some people.

In conclusion, Augmentin is an effective treatment for many types of bacterial infections. It is generally well-tolerated and has few side effects. However, it is not effective against all types of bacteria, and it can interact with other medications and cause allergic reactions in some people. Therefore, it is important to discuss the pros and cons of using Augmentin with your medical provider before starting treatment.

Preventative Measures to Avoid Bacterial Infections with Augmentin

Preventative measures are essential to avoiding bacterial infections and their associated complications. Taking augmentin, an antibiotic, can help prevent or reduce the severity of certain bacterial infections. However, there are many other preventative measures to consider when attempting to avoid bacterial infections. This book will discuss some of the most important preventative measures to avoid bacterial infections with augmentin.

The first preventative measure to take when attempting to avoid bacterial infections with augmentin is to practice proper hygiene. This includes regularly washing hands with soap and water, bathing regularly, and changing clothes and bedding as needed. Additionally, it is important to keep the home environment clean and free of bacteria. This may include regularly mopping and vacuuming, as well as disinfecting surfaces with a spray or disinfectant wipes.

The second preventative measure to take when attempting to avoid bacterial infections with augmentin is to get regular checkups and screenings. By getting regular checkups and screenings, any underlying conditions or infections can be identified and treated before they become more serious. Additionally, it is important to get vaccinated against common bacterial infections such as influenza, pneumonia, and meningitis. This can help reduce the risk of contracting these infections and any complications that may arise from them.

The third preventative measure to take is to eat a healthy, balanced diet. Eating a healthy diet that includes plenty of fruits, vegetables, and lean proteins can help maintain a strong immune system. Additionally, it is important to stay hydrated and get enough rest. This can help the body fight off any potential infections and reduce the risk of complications.

The fourth preventative measure to take is to avoid contact with people who are sick. This includes avoiding close contact with people who are coughing, sneezing, or exhibiting other signs of infection. Additionally, it is important to avoid touching surfaces that may be contaminated with bacteria. This includes doorknobs, handrails, and other objects that may carry bacteria.

The fifth preventative measure to take is to avoid overusing antibiotics. Overusing antibiotics can lead to antibiotic resistance, which can make treating bacterial infections more challenging. Additionally, it is important to only use antibiotics when prescribed by a doctor and to follow the instructions given carefully.

Finally, it is important to take any recommended supplements and medications. This includes taking any recommended Vitamin D, probiotics, and antibiotics such as augmentin. By taking recommended supplements and medications, the risk of contracting a bacterial infection can be reduced.

In conclusion, there are many preventative measures to take when attempting to avoid bacterial infections with augmentin. These include practicing proper hygiene, getting regular checkups and screenings, eating a healthy diet, avoiding contact with people who are sick, avoiding overusing antibiotics, and taking any recommended supplements and medications. By following these preventative measures, the risk of contracting a bacterial infection and its associated complications can be reduced.

CHAPTER FOUR

A Comprehensive Guide to Augmentin: Uses, Side Effects, and Interactions

Augmentin is a broad-spectrum antibiotic medicine that is used to treat bacterial infections of the skin, ears, sinuses and respiratory tract. It is a combination of amoxicillin and clavulanate potassium, which works together to inhibit the growth of bacteria. Augmentin is available in both a tablet form and a liquid suspension.

Augmentin is most commonly prescribed to treat bacterial infections such as bronchitis, sinusitis, and otitis media. It is also used to treat skin and soft tissue infections, such as boils and abscesses. In addition, Augmentin is sometimes prescribed for the treatment of urinary tract infections, pneumonia, and other more serious bacterial infections.

The most common side effects of Augmentin include nausea, vomiting, stomach pain, and diarrhea. Allergic reactions such as rash and hives are also possible. In more severe cases, Augmentin can cause liver and kidney damage. If you experience any of these side effects, contact your doctor immediately.

Augmentin can interact with several other medications. It is important to let your doctor know if you are taking any other medications, including birth control pills, antacids, or other antibiotics. Augmentin can also interact with certain foods, such as dairy products and alcohol, so it is important to avoid these while taking Augmentin.

Augmentin is not suitable for everyone. It should not be used by people who are allergic to amoxicillin or clavulanate potassium, or by women who are pregnant or breastfeeding. It is also not recommended for people with kidney or liver disease, or those with a history of jaundice or liver problems.

Before taking Augmentin, it is important to consult with your doctor to make sure it is the right medication for your condition. Your doctor can also provide you with any additional information on the side effects, interactions, and other important details about the medication.

It is also important to take Augmentin exactly as prescribed by your doctor. You should never take more or less than the recommended amount, and you should not take Augmentin for longer than your doctor has indicated. Additionally, you should always finish the entire course of medication, even if your symptoms seem to be improving.

If you have any other questions or concerns about Augmentin, it is important to discuss them with your doctor. Your doctor can provide specific instructions on how to take Augmentin safely and effectively. By following these instructions, you can reduce your risk of experiencing any of the side effects or interactions associated with the medication.

THE END

Printed in Great Britain
by Amazon

40873745R00030